# From Hell To Eternity

*A Journey Into The Last Days*

Written by, Anthony W. Antolic

© Antolic Enterprises 2017

ISBN-13: 978-0692784037

ISBN-10: 0692784039

# Preface

This journal was written by Anthony W. Antolic, as a means of both communication and trust between him and his wife. On September 6th, 2016; Tony learned that he had two years to live. He was given a chance to set right the things of his past. This journal is a day by day account of Anthony W. Antolic's last days among us.

By applying the restored gospel to both their lives, Tony and Kansa have been able to restore the health of a broken relationship, so they could face Tony's cancer together. By no means is Tony out of the woods, but his quality of life has improved a great deal.

This is a story of forgiveness and redemption. Anthony Wayne Antolic, has live the live most novelists would envy. "I have always been willing to try anything, if it would keep a roof over my families head." Anthony has always told those closest to him.

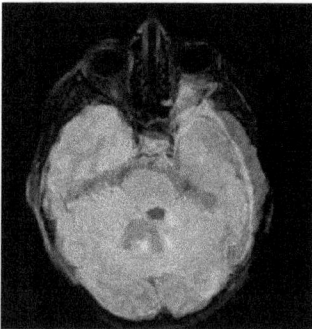

Anthony's diverse range of work experience has given him insights into his cancerous tumor that is expected to claim his life with in the next two years. Being the kind of man that doesn't know how to quit, Anthony started to research his own cure for his condition.

Tony's prognosis was 6 years ago, over 4 years longer than the so-called professionals told him that he would live. This day by day account of his trial and error approach to his own treatment is recorded in this journal.

Anthony's background in Anthropology gave him the starting point to succeed in defeating his silent enemy. But for Anthony total transparency is a major problem, so building trust has not been the easiest thing. In fact Anthony tends to use masks to disguise his true motives.

This day by day account of Anthony Antolic's  holistic  approach to defeating cancer was first written as a gift to his wife. He felt that Kansa would feel better if she knew all that he was doing to live a longer life. Anthony soon realized that this journal could help other win the fight so he took it more serious than just a daily journal. Anthony kept a record of scientific notes that could help advance cancer research as will as help others keep their marriage strong while dealing with these trials.

# CONTENTS

## My Addiction Almost Costed My Marriage

"God, grant me the serenity to accept the things I cannot change, Courage to change the things I can, And wisdom to know the difference" (American theologian Reinhold Niebuhr). The words are repeated at the beginning and end of every Addiction Anonymous meeting in America. Hello my name is not important, it should however be sufficient to say that I like many before me have hit rock bottom with my sex addiction when my wife left me. If was only for a short time but it was enough to realize that if I did not change I would be dying alone. I kept it from my wife for years but I have stage four cancer and the Doctors don't think that I will live to see my 45th birthday.

Needless to say, My drive to kick the addiction has never been stronger. I will never forget the night Kansa left. I was already feeling worthless because I could not do the job that I signed up for two days before.

# The Road Less Traveled

Sometimes we all must find away to turn the road less traveled into the well worn path. My life like many didn't start out well, but we all have the chance to end our race as the first through the finish line. In "Trials of the Heart[1], I talked about my

---

[1] Trails of the Heart ISBN-13: 978-1502538604

addiction to pornography and how I felt that I had a handle on it. Well I recently learned a valuable lesson about the need to avoid even the appearance of evil. To better explain, my wife Kansa left me for a brief time although it seemed like an eternity. It was really my secretive nature that made her feel that something was wrong. In fact I was hiding something from her that I probably shouldn't have. But before I tell you what this secret was, I must tell you a little bit about myself.

I spent my adult youth as a covert operative. I was raised in a family that moved around a lot and instead of trying to fit in I sat in the back of the class struggling with my school assignments. I never talked unless being spoken to and I never did anything to communicate other than answer questions. That's right I was not even trying to fit in. I viewed the popular kids as plastic dolls that needed to be broken and most of them liked to try to bully me. The foot ball team was the worst.

The Captain was always trying to get me to talk. One day he decided to throw a few punches at me in the middle of class. His friends joined in taking turns punching me in my kidneys and kicking me in the head. All the while my teachers stood by and did nothing and the other students cheered on their heroes. I new that the only way out of this was to make an example of the leader. I waited until he threw his next kick and I caught his foot and twisted his leg until I felt his ankle break as he screamed I kicked him in the balls over and over again but my objective was to end this bullying for good. The best way that I saw to do that was to make everyone involved understand that you never mess

You can find Trails of the Heart at:

https://www.amazon.com/dp/1502538601

with a Sheltiah knight. I broke both of his knees and his so-called friends were too scared to help him. This lack of courage was what I wanted the rest of my class to see.

"Hey punk where are your friends now? Look at them cowering in the corner like little girls. You are not as tough as everyone thought without your entire team behind you. That is ok because your football days are over." with that I severed his spine at his hip. Than I sat down and finished my assignment until the police came.

From that point on there was no bullying at Covington Jr High at least for that year. I got charged with assault but the entire student body gave their testimony in written form. I did have one more instant where some of the team sought revenge for their captain being put in a wheelchair but this time the student body joined together after I slammed a car door shut on the instigator's head.

I stayed at Covington for two more years and the time that I was there there was no fighting or even bullying. While an important event in my life, it was not my defining moment.

The event that truly defined me as what ever I am today happened when I was 12 years old, come to think of it, it was the same year as the fall of the Jr High royalty. Kelli and I were being made to have sex on film for her father's entertainment. One day in August of that year he had to answer a phone call and I told her it was time to escape. The whole time these words rushed through my head. "I will never surrender of my own free will. If in command, I will never surrender the members of my command while they still have the means to resist. If I am captured I will continue to resist by all means available. I will make every effort to escape and aid others to escape. I will accept neither parole nor special favors from the enemy."

We fled to my house and Author pulled some strings to get us state side. My grandfather helping us was in violation of a contract that merged the families together. All was fine until July 4th, 2001, when our car was hit head on by a drunk driver or so the story goes. All of my life I was told that my mission was to protect Kelliena from any and all potential threats. So I took her away from her father who was abusing her. I can't help but feel that my call costed her life. My wife Kansa felt that she was competing with Kelliena for my affection. I was not understanding what her concerns were about, until she walked out on me recently.

Kansa had left for about two weeks and it gave me an awakening that is slowly changing my life. One of her concerns was my temper. While I never hurt her I had a tendency to not only hurt the person who I perceived as a threat, I would also make sure that what what ever the person had that was making him a threat would be taken from him or her. In other words I was a person who was bent on Vengeance. Needless to say I was not a nice person. In fact I was a bit of a Jackass, to say the least.

I mean lets just recap what I have been talking about. In Junior High, I put one guy in a wheelchair and his friend in traction. I justified it with the fact that they were the school bullies, but lets get this straight: there is never any reason that any man has a right to let emotions get in the way of logic. I could have found another way to handle the football team, but the truth is I just didn't want too. I was out to hurt someone and end their football career. I let my anger at these guys fuel the pain I was going to make one of them feel until I took that pain away by breaking his back. I have a lot of regret about these things but I don't have time to relive the past. I am keeping this journal to help me know what I have to repent for.

Two weeks ago I was told by my doctor that I need to start getting my affairs in order. He told me that I had two years to live. Adult Gliomas, which I have been diagnosed with, may be highly aggressive, there may be pain and there is a very high mortality rate despite treatment. As a result I want to make amends to all the people who I may have wronged in the past. While I know that I can't undo the damage, at least I can try to acknowledge that I hurt these people and attempt to apologize.

No Jr. High School bully deserves to have his legs taken away just because I wanted to make an example of him. My sister may have been neglecting my nephew to the point that he was intentionally soiling his pants just so she would have to take the time to change his diaper at four years old, but I could have handled it so CPS did not take him out of the home. While her divorce was taking place. My biggest regret is that the last words I said to Author Nash were said in anger before he died.

I ran 20 miles that night because, I was so scared of what life would be like without my Grandfather. I don't even know when I got home or how. What I do remember was being so sore the next day that I could not move. I didn't say goodbye to even my girl friend and left a week later. I never told anyone where I went. I came back two years later and stayed for a month, only to leave again. I alienated every one around me and didn't seem to care.

I came back only to find out that my mother took it on her self to spit on her father's grave and invite the family pedophile into Author's house. I went to jail trying to defend my Grandfather's memory. My sister threw a punch at me and I reacted by opening my fingers and putting them through her ribs. I will never be sorry for this incident because I was up holding my Grandfather's wishes. In fact I was being nice because he told me to kill Mike Nash if for any reason he was to step foot onto Author's property. The time that I spent in jail gave my mother and sister the chance to take out a mortgage that they could not afford by putting my name down as a co-signer. My credit was destroyed even before I new what credit was. So I have my reasons for not having any contact with my family.

The sad part is now that I see the end, I hope that I can reconcile with them at least apologize for any wrongs. I am grateful that Tammie took me in, when I needed it but she needed a wake up call. Her son was perpetually crying and not even potty trained. His baby sitter was the television yet I became the bad guy?

At any rate, I am far from a saint. With the loss of my first wife, I went into hiding. I Literally joined a Catholic Monastery. When Author died I started running and I never stopped. Mount Angel Catholic Seminary was really just me running from things I was too afraid to face. Our marriage counselor asked me why I didn't stay in the Legion? Well the truth is the one skill that I mastered in my life besides using masks is running from my problems. That thing growing in my head is not so easy to run from. I left the Legion after having every bone in my body broken by Taliban Insurgents. I joined the Legion because I felt it would be 100% better than living in My Grandfather's house after my sister tricked her way into ownership. Besides without Author buffering the blows, those two women and I would have killed each other.

Doug asked me to write down anything that may keep me from an eternal life. Well it seems that I am apologizing for my existence. When I was 8 years old I took an oath that I hold firm too. This is the oath that I took.

"I am a knight of the Sheltiah order, fighting to guard my clan and our way of life. I am prepared to give my life in their defense.

I will never surrender of my own free will. If in command, I will never surrender the members of my command while they still have the means to resist.

If I am captured I will continue to resist by all means available and create further means for future resistance. I will make every effort to escape and aid others to escape. I will accept neither parole nor special favors [welfare] from the enemy. I accept that any governing authority out side of the Sheltiah community is not ordained by our creator and therefore is the enemy.

If I become a prisoner of war, I will keep faith with my fellow prisoners. I will give no information or take part in any action which might be harmful to my comrades. If I am senior, I will take command. If not, I will obey the lawful orders of those appointed over me and will back them up in every way.

When questioned, should I become a prisoner of war, I am required to take any opportunity to undermine my captors questions and further gather all forms of information that can be used against them in a counter strike. I will evade answering further questions to the utmost of my ability. I will make no oral or written statements disloyal to my oath or our allies or harmful to their cause.

I will never forget that I am a Sheltiah knight, fighting for freedom, responsible for my actions, and dedicated to the principles which keep my people free. I will trust in my God and in the wind that guides me, and the voice that harkins me." (The Oath of Shelta). I was made to memorize this as if it was scriptures.

At the same time I can't help but feel that God is using this trial to teach me a lesson in humility. Today is September 6th 2016. It has only been two weeks since my diagnosis and prognosis and I am seeing my health fail already. Kansa says that we are just more aware of it but the symptoms have been neglected for years. Anyway today I have had to deal with incontinence as well as projectile vomiting. I came home from work fixed Kansa and I dinner and for dessert a house that smelled of vomit. I tried to clean it up, only to add to the mess. I am being forced to depend on others for help and if this is God's way of teaching humility, I can't help but thing the it is cruel. If I am going to end up a Vegetable be for I meet Azrael on my way to Nog, I would rather die on my own terms. To be a burden on any one is not how I want to be remembered.

But suicide is not an option because of the oath that I hold so dear. I can not surrender the fight, neither can I accept help from a government whose Authority I neither recognize nor respect. Doug says that my accepting help from the Legion was using Tax dollars. But that is not how it works. If you did not earn the money for your health care you don't qualify, and American Taxpayers don't pay for the Legion in any way. France and her colonies put up the bill. So no Doug I don't, didn't, and never will ask for help from American Taxpayers. I had food stamps at one point in my life and fear that I never before committed such a heinous sin, as stealing from the sheep, while I should have been hunting wolves.

I was asked if I was ready to stand in judgment. The truth is there has never been a time in my life that I was not ready to die. I am ashamed of the fact that I had the chance to free America from the worst President in American History and did nothing. As a result countless innocent Americans have been lost as collateral damage in Obama's propaganda war.

On July 16th 1989, I attended my own funeral. On that day John Kelly Nash was given absolution for his transgressions because my unit understood that we may not be coming back. Our mission was to rescue an American politician from the Taliban. This mission unfortunately was successful and as a result the American people are living under Nazi rule. I accept the fate and consequences of my life choices. I ask forgiveness from those who I have wronged and as I am called out onto the carpet for the last time by the Lord of all creation, I do so with a spirit of truth repentance and humility. However, many of the things that I have fail to do has costed more lives than choosing the morally correct path at the time. If we would have just aborted the Mission Barack Obama would not have become president, and America would have been much better off.

On this last and final mission, failure is no longer a possibility it is a certainty. This mission is the one which everyone must embark. Some of us just know more about when.

09/09/2016

Today was my day off at LWO. Kansa and I need the money so I took a temporary job through Express. It was unloading a truck container by hand. Each box wade about 400 pounds and took two men to move it. My shoulder is toast right now. After work we went to see our marriage counselor. Doug got Kansa to open up to me about things that needed to be addressed. Earlier in our marriage we went to an adult theater where we both ended up doing things that hurt our relationship. I saw a side of my new wife that I didn't know was there. We both had sex with other people but Kansa went off the deep end. She had guys lining up to have their tern with my wife. It was as if she was pissing on my grave and I was not even dead. It was my idea to go there but Kansa was chomping at the bit to get there. This was a mistake that had us both acting out on our sex addictions. At any rate we agreed to go to our Bishop and confess our sins yet again. Kansa has been beating this dead horse ever since it happened.

We already confessed one of the incidents but every time we have a new Bishop the dirty laundry of our past has to be taken out of the rinse cycle before the dirt can be removed to be shown on the clothes line for all to see. We have to use the Atonement to do the rest. Kansa ended up in the psych ward more than once because of her inability to accept that the blood of Christ's Atonement would set us free if she would only have faith in its power.

10/09/2016

Kansa has made an appointment with the Bishop to talk about our transgressions that we have already talked about. We spent the day walking up and down the Art district of Portland and I priced CBD oil. Kansa has voiced that she feels helpless about the idea of my premature death but I have not given up. Research about Hemp oil has shown to not only ease pain but in some cases has reduced the size of the tumor.

The life I led before I came to the gospel was absolute filth. Group sex, pornography, and extortion was the norm. I want to clean up not only my spiritual life but my physical life as well. I have learned to appreciate my wife and honor our marriage in so many ways. Part of my new approach to life is cleaning up the mold in our apartment. After all clean living starts from the ground up.

Kansa and I have wanted to go on a vacation since we got married. Now it seems like we need to make some memories before I go to take my last ride with the ferryman. Our solution is a trip to Germany. We don't make a lot of money so we have to save for a while and cut back on things.

11/09/2016

01:19 hours, My shoulder still has not recovered from the work I did on Friday. My vision seems to be getting worse and I am dealing with incontinence of the colon. Last week I couldn't hold anything down and I must admit I am scared.

03:50 hours, up all night vomiting and dealing with a really rough case of diarrhea. I don't know if I am just sick or if this is part of having a really aggressive tumor in my brain. All that I do know is it is really hard to have faith in God's plan when dealing with this stuff. My mind is going 1000 miles a minute and none of it is good.

04:24 hours, My heart is beating out of my chest. I am not able to stay awake. My stomach muscles are so tight from the clinching that is feels likes I did 1000 sit-ups in an hour.

10:46 hours, stayed home from church to recover from a night of hell. As I lay my head back down and try to get some sleep, I am reminded of how blessed I have been to have Kansa in my life. The other day I had a vomiting fit that I was too sick to clean up. After Kansa made sure I was going to be alright she cleaned up the mess not once but twice. She always goes the extra mile and I am a better man because of it. At this point I don't know if I can make it to work tomorrow but I will try. I do it for Kansa. After all marriage is about a dedication to sacrifice for your partner: we must always remember that lust is destructive but a loving sacrificial devotion to each other is eternal.

13:00 hours, I am feeling better. Kansa is still at church and I think we are going to be excommunicated from the church for stuff that we already dealt with years ago, because Kansa has to keep bringing it up as if it was a new event. All I can say is Mormons are almost as strange as Democrats. I have to get something to eat. I pray that this time I can hold it down.

Kansa and I were sealed in the Temple and I plan to make good on that promise. Kansa had a good meeting with the Bishop.

22:47 hours, Kansa and I are at odds with her family's meddling in our marriage. She keeps saying that they only had a her best interest in mind. But the way they did it would have had us divorced in another week, and I know that was what they felt was what they felt was in my wife's best interest. I know that Kansa needs her family because of the way she was raised, but I don't know how to forgive them for the game they played in all of this. For Kansa's sake I know I need to find away.

12/09/2016

I don't know how to keep the faith when the body of believers that are closest to me almost destroyed both Kansa and my life. To be under the control of any person other than the one who created you is not God's will. Kansa's family took her phone away and when she asked for it back they refused. She was a prisoner to the will of who ever would give her a ride and she would not have been aloud to talk to me even if she wanted to while she was in the custody of her family. Her fear was she would not be allowed to stay where she was if she did not obey the rules. Thus she truly was not acting on her own free will. I have the medical power of attorney for my wife so according to the Prosecutor I had a case for kidnapping. I did not pursue it because that would have hurt our relationship even more.

Still I need to find away to look passed their involvement and move on. I only have a short time with Kansa and I need it to be happy. I refuse to be that kid I was in Junior High. Some how I need to work passed this and just accept they were trying to help. I am not sure if I can or even want to, though. It has become apparent to me the at least one Mormon family ignores the scriptures, Genesis 2:24, Ephesians 5:31, Matthew 19:5, that all say, "For this reason a man will leave his father and mother and be united to his wife, and the two will become one flesh." "I have seen some women who give their children that spot, that preeminence, in their affection and crowd out the father. That is a serious mistake." (Ensign, Mar. 1976, p. 72.) seems how every member of Kansa's family has made this same mistake and been through several divorces themselves, they should probably, "take the plank out of their own eyes before trying to take the speck out of mine" (Matthew 7:5).

None of us are perfect, least of all me. I have destroyed lives in the name of justice. My shot has changed the course of history and not always for the better. Many times I have had to regret letting the wrong person live. The blood of my teammates are on my hands and I don't sleep well at night. Every day I ask God for his forgiveness and grace to help me through. My biggest issue is learning to forgive myself. My faith wavers with the good days and the bad. My Bishop told me that I will never learn to forgive others until I learn to forgive myself..

Only three days after Kansa left me my mother in-law sent me this Email pretending to be my wife:

> "Dear Tony, This is Kansa! I want you know that I love you and want to work on mending our relationship! It is my belief in order to heal our relationship you must agree to a formal separation and have a third party counselor work with us to improve our relationship. I believe that this absolutely necessary for us to rebuild. I know we both have problems that need to be addressed. I need to be assured that you will not come looking for me, so that I can have the freedom to do what needs to be done. We will communicate through a third party advocate, i.e... Family member, Bishop, counselor etc. I believe this is the only way and path to heal [The lack of punctuation told me this was not my wife.]"

I knew it was not Kansa because I know My wife and I highlighted the inconsistency that saved our marriage. Kansa never uses the explanation point for anything. She would have never used "i.e." in her writing and the use of the term formal separation stunk like the modeling of Kansa's parents. I filled out the divorce papers and promised myself that if Lana kept trying to control me and Kansa I would file for divorce. After Kansa came home I showed he the text and she denied writing it. But she did tell me that her mother and Jim talked about what to say with her as they drove to the temple. My wife would have never texted me about something so important. She always said that would be rude.

However, if she was going to let her mother continue manipulating like children to the point that she would agree to a formal separation after only three days I was not going to play the game. I was done. No one was listening. I knew I didn't have the Time that every one wanted to give. Both Lana and Jim lied to my face and I was to trust them? Wow! Mormons are weird.

# From Hell To Eternity
Written by Anthony W. Antolic

## Staying Active Keeps My Depression At Bey.
13/09/2016

I am pleased to report that Kansa found a job at a bowling alley down the street. I am happy in the warehouse at LWO. Today was just a good day. Kansa will more than likely be working a swing shift but it is so close to the house that she can walk.

11:34 hours, Kansa is saying goodbye to he friends at AWC. She starts her new job tomorrow. Tonight I have the Boy Scouts. But for some reason the Day is dragging for me. The took me out of the warehouse and put me on the floor. I am standing here sanding parts. And I am so board I am falling asleep.

I got through the work day and came home long enough to go the a boy scout  I have not been involved with the Boy Scouts since may of 2016. But my shift changed from swing to days and now I can get involved again. It is good to feel needed. I have needed ways to serve to help me keep my mind off of the fact that I probably will not see these boys graduate.

14/09/2016

I got home from work just in time to kiss Kansa goodbye. Today she started her new job at the bowling alley down the street. My biggest fear at this point is that Kansa will leave me again. Everyone kept telling me that she needs time. Well I don't have time. At least I don't have time for childish games. I eat a diet of vegetables and water with practically no animal proteins. I cook everything in CBD oil because I read that tumors have been reduced or even healed by using Hemp oil. I pray to my creator, saying thank you for letting me have one more day with my wife. I plan to walk down to Kansa's new job every day to walk with her back home. It is the little things that make memories. If the Lord takes me before Kansa, I plan to give her no reason to doubt that I love her and will for the rest of time.

21:43 hours, I have decided not to stay on this Vegetables diet. With every day that has passed, I have lost energy. I am a carnivore. Vegetables are what you feed live stock upgrade to a steak dinner. The diet I was on had me dreading the next meal and I couldn't eat enough. If I am going to stay active and enjoy my time with Kansa, then I need to feel like. Something more than a walking corpses.

How you do on certain diets has a lot to do with your blood type. The R.H. factor can tell you if it would be a good idea to become a vegetarian. For example, I have O- blood. Meaning I have not genetic material from the Rheses monkey. What it also means is that I have been eating right for my blood type my entire life.

"O" type and that all humans at one time maintained this blood group before the subsequent evolutionary appearance of blood types A, B and AB (reference 1, pp. 6-13). Accordingly, Peter believes that people with the O blood type had ancestors who were skillful hunters and whose diets were high in meat and animal proteins. For modern people with the O blood type he advocates a high meat, low carbohydrate "hunter" diet, with virtually no wheat, few grains or legumes and limited dairy products.

15/09/2016

21:30 hours, I fell asleep only to wake up to an empty bed. I had forgotten that Kansa is working swing now. Every fear of the passed month came back to me. I walked to the bowling alley, just for my selfish need to know that she was just at work and didn't abandon me again. I was planning to make the trek just to get out of the house. But this time was more for peace of mind than the Exercise. I love her so much and I need her to return that love.

16/09/2016

I made it through another week, but Kansa is struggling with the stress from her new job. I have to go and print up her food handlers card as soon as the Library opens. I pray that she can make this work. This job is much more than just an income for her it is teaching her to become more independent and self-confident. These are both qualities that she will need when I am gone. I am going to walk down to the bowling alley in a few minutes to check on her. After that I need to go to work myself. Every day I pray that God will give us on more day to be together.

I need Kansa much more than She needs me, although she thinks it is the other way around. I have started to do Tia-Chi before I go to bed at night. I feel a bit better every day but in the back of my mind I still can't dismiss the words of my doctor. "Mr. Antolic, you need to get your affairs in order." But I'll talk about that after work. By the way after the CBD pills I have not vomited once. I am still taking 1500 mg of Vitamin C three times a day. I know that Kansa and I can beat this. And I thank God for this chance to turn my life around.

11:00 hours, Justin called and told me not to go in to work, he does not have the overtime budget.

13:35 hours, Kansa was sent home from the bowling alley. She was concerned about my laying into her, but when I went to she her she was clearly out of her element. My biggest issue is making sure that Kansa is safe and happy. So I took her out to a movie and told her to quit her job. She was so relieved. Now we are in for the night.

Kansa would have stayed just to make my sorry butt happy, however my need to see her happy can sometimes cause issues in our relationship. Kansa and I had a large communication issue about my tumor. I wanted to protect her and did nothing to tell her about it. This ultimately led to her thinking that I way cheating on her when in fact I way going to doctors. This caused her to leave me for a brief time that seemed like an eternity. I made a promise to her and myself that I would not hold anything back ever again.

We fight more but at least we are talking. When deception is apart of a relationship the relationship is bond to fail.

23:09 hours, well it is time to hit the sack. Kansa is already asleep and I am done for the day.

18/09/2016, 08:04 hours:

Today is Sunday. For a Mormon Sundays mean 3hours in church and other activities that keep the Sabbath holly. I never understood the concept of treating one day different than all the rest. I mean frankly the cows on a farm who were also create by God don't know that it is Sunday. They still need to be feed and milked. So how is it that the Pharisees and Sadducees could interpret the day of rest as a day that they could not take more then ten steps? Staying Active is a fundamental part of staying healthy so something had to be lost in the interpretation. The

Mormons view the Sabbath as a day of service rather than a day of rest. Take time to visit someone who is sick and even fixing someone's car so they can get to work the next day is viewed as keeping the Sabbath holly. Today I plan to invite a homeless couple over to dinner.

But the Sabbath should not be an excuse to live a righteous life. The games that we play and the words that we say should always be a reflection of our Savior's love for us.

## Keeping A Balance Of All Aspects Of Our Lives

08:51 hours, yesterday my attitude had to change when I saw that Kansa was trying as hard as she was at the bowling alley and her health was getting in the way. I have noticed the same thing happening in my life and I have to reevaluate my stand on the idea of government assistance for the disabled.

I am a Veteran of three wars and the men I survived would gladly shoot themselves in the head before asking for help even after the loss of a limb. But I have more than just me to concern myself with, now I am responsible for Kansa and the Misfit mindset must be pushed aside. Its funny to me, but I have been on this earth for 42 years and I am still learning about the world around me.

11:06 hours:

Up till now, religion has been a tool to understand and manipulate the people around me, but now as the saying goes, "there are no Atheists in foxholes." I thank the Lord for having Kansa drag me to church all the times I didn't want to go.

Kansa voiced a need for me to be honest with her about everything. Well my holding things back could have destroyed our marriage, so honesty is the way to go.

22:03 hours:

Kansa and I had a flight about the fact that her family did everything they could to destroy our marriage.

19/09/2016, 21:10 hours:

I have noticed that a positive attitude towards live in general has a profound impact on my physical well being. I woke up in a bad mood today and soon after came migraines and vomiting. The CBD pills have curbed that for the most part and the Vitamin C has helped give me back my Energy. However, a simple attitude adjustment can change all of that. I just got done watching a DVD called "The Secret," it talks about how our negative emotions can attract more negative events. I would recommend everyone watches this video.

I have put myself onto a regiment of drinking a glass of water with four drops of Hydrogen peroxide in it daily. I heard about people successfully killing cancer in their bodies with this technique. I figure I am dead anyway so what could it heart. It tastes bad but if it works, I am grateful.

Still the balance between spiritual and physical must be met. This may be the toughest fight of my life, but as any boxer will tell you, "if you find yourself in the corner you don't give up, that is when you fight even harder."

20/09/2016, 05:30 hours:

If you read any of my other books, then you know that I struggle with a porn addiction. However, life got much easier once I was able to separate the meaningless act of sex from making love to my wife. I don't have time for arguing about why she doesn't trust me. All I want is to spend my time that I have left making memories that Kansa will want to revisit. I need to know that when we part ways that Kansa would be proud to say that I am her husband.

22:08 hours:

If it was not for the fact that I can talk to my phone to type. I would not be making this entry. The migraines just keep coming. I vomited at work today and they almost sent me home. Kansa has been a real trooper through all of this. I went to my Boy Scout meeting and was glad I did. Still everything hurts and I wish it would end. If I am as dizzy as I am in the morning I may have to call in.

05:30 hours:

I did end up calling in. I am concerned about how the night went. I kept waking up trying to breath. The migraine still has not let up and under the stress I am temped to act out on my sex addiction. I refuse to give in though. I did not get any sleep so that is going to be my next attempt. I think what vexes me the most is that defeat seems like the only outcome for this battle.

After going to urgent care, got same same song and dance. "We can give you something for the pain Mr. Antolic, but at this point we are not set up to help you. I went home and took my CBD pill and went to sleep. My faith in modern medicine has never been lower.

18:45 hours:

I took five drops of Hydrogen Peroxide in a 16 once glass of water with some lemon juice and honey, to choke it down. I do this three times a day with the Vitamin C and CBD caps. Then Kansa and I went to Win-Co for some odds and ends. I am praying that my heart well calm down in time to go to work in in the morning.

I had to tell my boss about the tumor today and I am nervous about the outcome.

22/09/2016, 16:21 hours:

I have learned to take the good days with the bad. Yesterday, I could not walk across the room without puking. Today I am on top of the world. I put in a full day at work and came home and make dinner. I thank God for every day that I have and think of it as a gift. My name may have been plucked from the tree of life and the Angel of Death my be waiting in the wings to take me off the stage before the final act, but at least today I have lived a fruitful and productive life.

21:56 hours:

Kansa is a sleep and my Dad finally texted me back, after weeks of trying. The Mormons believe that family is forever. Well that would not be a selling point when talking about most of my family. However, Kansa's family is extremely important to her and I envy that.

23/09/2016, 02:15 hours:

Kansa wants me to be what Doug likes to call transparency. I know that I have compromised her trust, but to have outsiders involved in our lives is against all that I was raised to believe. Still I have to be accountable to someone other than myself. Otherwise my self destructive nature would destroy me.

In a nutshell my wife wants to know if I have ever been unfaithful to her. Well let me just say that the only times I have been with anyone other than Kansa was with Kansa's consent, in a group sex scenario. We both regret the decision. As I face my own mortality, I pray that others can learn from my many mistakes.

I have bought into the words concepts of morality to justify my bad choices. In my frustration with my own personal regrets my own natural man tends to over power my judgement. My concern for the consequences for my actions become void and the objective of the moment is all that is relevant. At least that is where I am coming from.

I do believe that through the acceptance of the Atonement, I know that I can and will change. Kansa is the only person who I let into my life. Unfortunately my past decisions have forced others into my world without being invited. For this reason I can and will not be able to forgive myself.

I have never cheated on my wife! Yet she chooses to believe otherwise because my private nature has never allowed me to seek out interaction with others. I have been able to let Kansa into my life more than even my first wife or my Grandfather. Yet at the same time I have not been able to let her completely into my life. This fact has worked against me as I have lost control of my addiction to pornography and sought after things that were far less gratifying than the simple act of holding Kansa as she goes to sleep. I talk more about my addiction in "Trails of the Heart," but I don't think Kansa has ever read any of my books. Sad, because they are truly me pouring my heart out to Kansa in the only from of communication that I have that will not me clam up once I start interacting with people.

Before the tumor became noticeable, I could glance at a page once and never have to look at it again. I would read it when I was talking to someone. Now I have to look at the same page a dozen times and still not get what is was saying. The vision in my good eye is starting to fail and I am dropping things at work. Still

I know in my heart that I will beat this and live a long and fruitful life with the one person who I trust enough to let into my world.

In general I hate people. But Kansa has this innocents about her that makes me feel safe. Most of the time, I meat someone and I go through phases, that determine whether or not I would need to kill them latter. I even run through the pattern that would get me to the end game fastest. While all of that is going on in my head I may be having a polite conversation with them. I never had to do that with Kansa. She had my heart from our first conversation. The fact that my actions pushed her out of my life, scares me more than death. Let my routing coupes pollute the street. I don't give a rat's ass. Just don't take the one person who has ever mattered to me walk away. I told Kansa that I don't deny any thing that she accuses me of, because she already made up her mind about the issue. I wonder why she even stays around because I can tell her the truth and in her mind I am lying her unless she hears what ever it is that she wants to hear. My heart has broken.

I don't given a damn about reconciliation with the Bishop. I am a cold blooded killer and by definition I know I am going to Hell, so why bother with the steps of reconciliation. I remember the face of every target. The orders given and the all clear to fire the shot. They all had families that I destroyed with my trigger. I can't forgive me so why would Jesus? Kansa concerns herself with my addiction to porn and justified it is I still see the blood of the man I just shot spraying all over his teenage daughter. How can that be forgiven?

I pray every night for the forgiveness of Chris. The nightmares don't happen as often but they still do. Yet Kansa is worried about porn? I still hear my spotter in the background saying, "hold the shot!". But it was too late. The trigger pulled and an innocent man fell to the ground and my wife is concerned with porn?

I love Kansa and I never want to hurt her again. I pray the my death be swift and quiet, so she can get on with her life. The is no reconciliation for the death of an innocent. So after this life we will be parted. I just wish God would hurry up.

There has been no infidelity on my party. I have talked to people on the chat line knowing that like me they are all talk and would never hook up with anyone. In fact you give them your address and they back out of the conversation. That is the rules of the game. But at know time was I ever thinking about meeting up this them. This is not an excuse, I just was not looking at the whole picture. If I was Kansa I would be thinking I was being unfaithful too. After all "if you lust after a woman in your heart, you have already committed adultery" (Matthew, 5:28).

08:52 hours:

Kansa is a sleep at my side. I want to go onto record as to say that Kansa can use or look through my phone at any time. I feel that it is an invasion of privacy but I have nothing to hide from the only person in this life that matters to me. However, if Kansa's family ever gets involved in our marriage again, I will be the one to leave and Kansa will not have to concern herself with what to do with my body. Her betrayal on this matter can not be repeated. If I learned of another occurrence I would not be will to live another day. My funeral will be simple and I don't care about what any law of a dead government has to say about it. I have stuffed my Sunday suite with 25 pounds of Magnesium. Kansa has heard me say that I wouldn't be caught dead in a pare of slacks an a sport coat. Well here is. a my sense of irony.

When I get to become a burden on anyone I plan to drive out to the beach where sand can't catch fire so the flames will be contained and put on the suite and cover myself in gas and strike a match. At over 3000° F not even the bone will remain. Kansa will have no fine Expenses and the dead will be done. No one should ever be allowed to get so involved in another man's life that even the way we are allowed to die is regulated. This will be my Final act of rebellion against a government that has fooled generations into thinking they are free.

But don't give up on me yet. I still have some fight left in me. I am planning to live lone passed the doctor's time line just because he told me what would happen with my life. I have to out live him just to take a crap on his grave and say I told you so.

But why do that Doctors don't have any concern for you but they will take your money.

09:54 hours:

Next week I am taking Kansa up to see my father. He knows about the Tumor but not the prognosis. Kansa is still sleeping and never has there been a sweeter Angel. Anyway, it is time for breakfast.

25/09/2016, 01:19 hours:

I feel betrayed by Kansa's family. A while back, Kansa left me. She said that she wanted to work things out. But her family took her phone away. Then her mom texts me posing as Kansa and tells me that I would have to agree to a formal separation. I have never seen a formal separation result in anything but divorce. Family should never be involved with marital spats. If Lana would have written less professionally and I believed that it was Kansa writing it. I would have just filed for a divorce. After all it was only a few days in and she had not talked to me at all and the only thing I get is a request for a filing for a separation. It became clear to me that Kansa's family had been manipulating both of. us.

Soon after that I started getting messages from Kansa's friends asking why she had not answered her messages. That is when I knew that her family had taken her phone. So as far as I knew she had no car and would be a prisoner to the will of her captors and her phone was taken away. Because Kansa has a history of mental illness she is easier to control than most and Clark County's Prosecutor was ready to press charges against Tim and Airy Godfrey as well as Jim and Lana Hill. His angle was that I am the holder of Kansa's Medical Power of Attorney and there were ample people voicing concern to the Police to file a missing persons report that would become Kidnapping charges.

Here was my concern. Kansa has been known to go manic and just start wondering the streets. With her cell phone turned off I had no choice but to assume that her battery died and she was not wanting to seek shelter. History has seen this before. Nicole Davis a Prosecutor for Clark County, asked me if I felt she was being unlawfully held against her will. I told her that she is probably going to say it is of her own free will but once she realizes that she was not free to come and go or talk to the outside word she would change her story. Mis Davis asked me to bring Kansa in when I get a chance. We are going in on Wednesday.

25/09/2016, 11:26 hours:

Last night I learned that the one interaction between Kansa and I while she left was a fraud. It was a text that. Claimed it was Kansa when in fact Kansa admitted it was her Mom writing it.

Due to the use of the words formal separation after only a few days, I had to consider the Idea of going straight to a divorce. But then I realized that Kansa did not write the text. I was not important enough to tell me that she was wanting to go before a judge and get officially separated. So instead she had her mother text it to me.

After last night I am wondering if I even want Kansa around. I know that I screwed up and I deserve to burn in Hell. I have held my ticket for years, but for brief moments in time I was happy but then Kansa's family got involved. I wish I could just let this go and forgive everyone but all I want to do is crawl into a ball and wait to die. I will not be seeing Doug anymore. Why bother. My calling at church is taken care of and all I plan to do is go to work to take care of someone who didn't seem to think I was important enough to even communicate with until the Reaper takes me. If the Doc is right and I pray that he is, it will not be long now. The one thing I pray who every is reading this will take from this is that families may be important but they should never be involved in the marriage between two people. I was given paperwork from my boss to apply from a medical leave. I am not going to take it. In fact I am hoping that I drop a load and kill myself. It would put an end to this constant pain and no one would miss me anyway.

I can't stop thinking about these negative thoughts. I stayed home from church because I feel like my world has crumbled down around me and why in the hell should I care about a soul that was forfeit years ago? As far as I know that Atonement does not apply to murder. I can't stop hearing that 16 year old girl's scream as her father fell to the ground. Just as my hand squeezed, I heard my spotter yell out, "Hold the SHOT!". Like Kansa says, I just can't let it go.

I was cleared and the finds said that we had bad intel, but I don't know how to let it go. I have pushed everyone out of my life, because I don't feel worthy of happiness. On the other hand, this journal off e rs me a place to vent and now I now what I need to do. If I leave now the classes may be over and the Bishop will be having the meeting with Kansa and the endless apologizing for things we already talked about. At the same time I can't keep my eyes opened and I just want to sleep.

26/09/2016, 22:15 hours:

Kansa called her Mom and finally told her to but out of our marriage. I am not keeping her from her family but both Lana and Jim, Kansa's parents flat out lied to me to my face and I don't have time for liars. So Kansa told her that any discussion about our marriage is off limits. In other news Kansa and I got a hold of my father and we are going to see him on Saturday. I have not seen him for over half of my life time. I am a bit nervous. Kansa asked her Mom why she would pretend to be Kansa to ask me for a formal separation. I have never seen a separation not end in divorce.

I took one of the CBD pills this morning to kill a migraine. It did not help. I had to work park of the morning out in the Sun. The migraine will be gone by morning but they seem to be coming more often.

Today I fell at work but no one saw, so it is fine. Work, Church and family time is all that I have left. I must learn to forgive. I can't emphasize enough how important the scriptures have become in our lives.

27/09/2016, 16:45:

I don't remember much about the day. My boss, Justin took my home after having a Seizure. Yet, some how I ended up at the Library. I texted Kansa because I couldn't remember how to get home.

Being at home gave me time to do some research. A friend sent me a video that opened my eyes.[2] For years I blamed myself for the death of an innocent man. My friend was my spotter during the operation. I realized that I was a pawn in a game that was being played on the international stage. I had no responsibility for my orders or why they were given. It was my last mission with the Legion. I was assigned to a nearby roof top on 20 October 2011, officially I was no longer with the unit but they needed someone who was not going to be recognized, because my unit trains in Libya.[3] I was still on reserve status and they put me in the field.

The objective was a 69 year-old man who was being held by National Transitional Council forces. He was being moved with a bag over his head. Now I had not been in Libya since 1988 and I don't watch the news. So I did not question the order to make the shot until the blood sprayed and the girl next to him took the bag from his head. The NTC initially claimed, he died from injuries sustained in a firefight when loyalist forces attempted to free him. Stories and videos would be released to the public of his last moments that show rebel fighters beating him and one of them sodomizing him with a bayonet, before he was shot

---

[2] This is the link to the video:

https://youtu.be/hHMeONfUXNg

[3] Kansa was spending a week with her family on a campout.

several times as he shouted for his life. However with the black bag over his head anyone could say that the prisoner was Muammar Gaddafi.

Think about this, why would there by a video of the invasion of a compound and the beating and killing of a prisoner, during a firefight, unless it was staged?

It is my belief that I or anyone else for that matter, doesn't have time to harbor ill will towards others. None of us are perfect. My wife and her family pulled our marriage out and plastered it on a billboard. Yet, thanks to the invasion of our privacy, we are talking. We are going to see my Dad in two days and we are working pay off as much of our bills, while we still can. Forgiveness is my biggest challenge. I know that none of us are perfect, least of all me. If I have wronged anyone in any way, I want to make amends.

I grew up being told that my father would beat me and abuse me in other ways. As an adult I realized the much of that was the product of a bitter woman who never wanted his kids to see him again. After my father contacted me to tell me that he was not dead I contemplated telling Kansa the whole story about the fake death certification.

My grandfather put a price on my father's head. I forged the Death Certificate to protect him. But that is not a skill that good Mormons talk about. I pray that the people I have wronged can find peace in this life or the next.

29/09/2016, 22:51 hours:

I was raised to question every aspect of Authority. This is not always a good idea. But my instincts have me asking basic questions. For example if you can't cut into my head to biopsy the tumor, how can you say that I only have two years to live? The sad fact is that Doctors like the rest of us are not Gods. The are going to work everyday like the rest of us.

So all Dr. Kevin Braxton M.D. has to go on is passed history. But I am a fighter. I refuse to buy into the prognosis and just give up on life. Although I admit some days it would be that much easier. The Peroxide Therapy and CBD pills seem to work but not if my attitude is that of a quitter. Having Kansa at my side has been a wonderful gift from God. She has proven that she meant the words for better or for worse. I promise her that I will never give up. And the promise keeps me going some days. Still I feel God's grace working in hour lives.

## Marriage is a Sacrifice

I can't tell you how much I took my wife for granted. I never realized how much Kansa did for me on a daily basis, until she walked out. The Christian rock group "Casting Crowns." has a song called, "Broken." The Chorus of the song says "let's be broken together." Will that is Married life for Kansa and I.

We both have our faults and we choose to live with them out of love for the other person. I regret that I took Kansa leaving me to realize that I had to give up my private life to let someone into the screwed up world life that has chosen me. It is 22:52 hours and this incredible journey is coming to an end for one more day. Kansa is asleep and I packed her lunch for work tomorrow.

My day is going to change a great deal as the Seizure at work means I will not be driving the forklift. Still like everyone else, I go to work as a Sacrifice for my family so we have a roof over head and food on the table. But we both make sacrifices for our marriage. Kansa asked me to get ride of the rated "R" movies. That meant getting ride of a childhood favorite. I am going to miss watching "Stripes." Have a good night.

30/09/2016, 18:20 hours:

Tomorrow Kansa and I go to visit my father. He is planning to take us to a local casino for brunch. Today went well at work and I have been thinking about marketing this journal. It is my belief that passing on what I have learned could help others.

As my wife and I deal with our individual health conditions, we find that the basic skill of budgeting our finances is increasingly important. We both work for an hourly wage and if we are unable to be at work, our budget for the month suffers.

My boss approved my application for the Oregon state Medical Leave Act. What this means is my job is protected should I not be able to make it in to work due to my health. I don't get paid for the time but at least we know I will still have a job if or when things get bad.

22:56 hours:

The seasons have changed. Summer has come and gone, and Autumn has begun to paint the leaves on the trees. I love this time of years. But the change of seasons this years marks the turning of the tide in our marriage. Our future is not as certain as it once was.

Kansa has been asked to clean up my vomit and. Tolerate my mood swings. This is too much to ask of anyone. Yet she is here and willing to do these things. Love is a dedication to your partner.

## From Hell To Eternity
Written by Anthony W. Antolic

# About The Author

Anthony Wayne Antolic has always been a fighter. He faced combat in the deserts of the middle east and the flood waters of Hurricane Katrina. He learned to read and made his way through college as an adult. Now he has to face rebuilding his marriage, cancer and a full time job while he sees the tumor in his head taking his sight. The Doctor's may have given up but the former Legionare never learned how to quit. This is his journal that was written in the hope that his success and failure can offer hope to others.

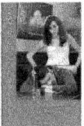

Trails of the Heart "Why is America Addicted to our Addictions?"

Trails of the Heart gets its name from the fact that even the smallest sin can effect others. This book looks at the Addiction recovery process from a christian point of view. It asks the question, "if Americans had control over our addictions, could our economy survive?"

ISBN-13: 978-1502538604

Publication Date: May 14, 2015

Language: English

Number of Pages: 116

The Road To Salvation "Because With God We Prosper &
Without Him We Fail!!!"

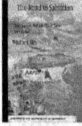

You may have noticed a steady trend of moral
decline, religious indifference, increasing crime as
well as unemployment. Could the Supreme Court's
ruling that defines the First Amendments separation
of Church and State clause in 1972 have contributed to these
trends? Is it possible that many of the human trends are being
intentionally designed to corrupt the American understanding of
freedom? If so, who benefits?

ISBN-13: 978-1329300200

Publication Date: August 1, 2015

Language: English

Number of Pages: 288

# From Hell To Eternity
Written by Anthony W. Antolic

## Notes & Bibliography

1. The hactivist group known as Anonymous, exposed the truth about Chemotherapy.

2. CBD oil: "Simply put, cannabinoids are naturally occurring compounds found in the cannabis plant. There are dozens of compounds including Cannabidiol (CBD), THC, and a host of other cannabinoids. Together they are responsible for the benefits and drawbacks to medical marijuana and industrial hemp-based products." https://healthyhempoil.com/cannabidiol/

3. Hydrogen peroxide therapy: a few drops of Hydrogen Peroxide in water once a day is said to have worked to cure cancer by burning out the tumor. If you start vomiting you are taking too much.[4]

4. Blood Type Diet: The blood type diet is based on your personal blood type. It is easier than most because your body craves what the diet calls for anyway.

5. Pistachios and other nuts have the nutrients that can help fight cancer.

6. I have learned that my attitude can mean the difference between a day filled with pain and a life of memories.

---

[4] I am not a medical Doctor, these are things that I have tried to improve my quality of life.

7.   Muammar Gaddafi's death was just another flag that the Magician flies to distract you. Satan uses distraction to hide his true intentions.

8.   You can find more of Anthony W. Antolic's books at: http://www.Amazon.com/author/anthonyantolic

9.   While Kansa and Anthony were separated their marriage counselor had them only communicating by Letters and Facebook Messenger. By having to take the time to write, the couple was forced to think about the words that would be written.

# From Hell To Eternity

Written by Anthony W. Antolic

Published by Antolic Enterprises

© 2017, Antolic Enterprises.

1414 NE Minnehaha Street, Vancouver WA. 98665 (USA)

+1 (360) 932-1315

Written by, Anthony and Kansa Antolic

Edited by,

$12.00
ISBN 978-0-692-78403-7
51200>

www.ingramcontent.com/pod-product-compliance
Lightning Source LLC
Chambersburg PA
CBHW060530280326
41933CB00014B/3123

# FACTS AND TRIVIA ON AMERICA'S MOST HEATED PRESIDENTIAL RIVALRY

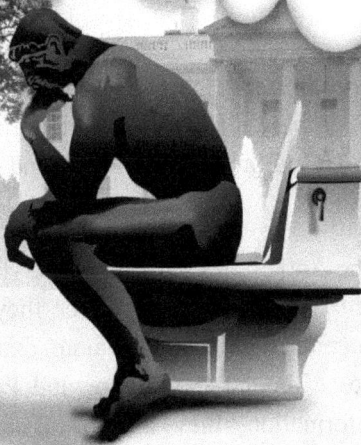

**Learn America's future in 20 minutes**

With Bern Bolo
The Bathroom Genius